Life with Wellbeing

Grace White

Grace White

Legal and legal data
Copyright holder: © Sebastian MG
Author: © Grace White
Year: 2024

Index

Introduction to Wellbeing

Wellbeing is a broad concept that covers various aspects of our lives, from physical to emotional and mental health. In essence, it is about feeling good about yourself and your environment. Having well-being does not simply mean being free of disease, but rather living in a way that promotes optimal quality of life. Wellbeing is about balancing the different aspects of our lives so that we can enjoy each day to the fullest and face challenges with resilience.

Imagine waking up every morning with energy, motivation, and a sense of purpose. This is possible when we take care of our health as a whole. Well-being starts with diet, exercise, sleep and stress management. But it goes beyond the physical. It also includes our relationships, our emotions, our environment, and how we feel about ourselves. Everything is interconnected. When one part of our life is out of balance, it can affect the others.

Food plays a fundamental role in our well-being. What we eat not only affects our physical health, but also our mood and energy. Eating a balanced and nutritious diet provides us with the necessary nutrients to stay active and healthy.

Including a variety of fruits, vegetables, proteins, and whole grains in our diet can make a big difference in how we feel day to day.

Exercise is another pillar of well-being. It's not just about maintaining a healthy weight, but about moving our body to release tension, improve our mood, and strengthen our muscles and bones. You don't have to be a professional athlete to benefit from exercise. Simple activities like walking, dancing, or practicing yoga can have a significant impact on our health and happiness.

Sleep is the third crucial component of well-being. A good rest is essential for the repair and regeneration of our body and mind. Without enough sleep, we feel tired, irritable, and less able to cope with daily challenges. Establishing a regular sleep routine and creating an environment conducive to rest can help us improve the quality of our sleep and, consequently, our general well-being.

Managing stress is essential to maintaining well-being. Stress is an inevitable part of life, but when it becomes chronic, it can have negative effects on our health. Learning relaxation techniques, such as meditation, deep breathing and mindfulness, can help us reduce stress and improve our quality of life. Additionally, taking time for ourselves, doing things we enjoy, and connecting with our loved ones can also be very beneficial.

Emotional health is equally important. Recognizing and managing our emotions, both positive and negative, allows us to live in a more balanced way. Practicing gratitude, self-care, and seeking support when we need it are key strategies for maintaining good emotional health. We should not be afraid to express our emotions or ask for help when we need it.

Our relationships also play a crucial role in our well-being. Having meaningful connections with family, friends, and the community provides us with support, love, and a sense of belonging. Open communication, empathy and respect are essential to building and maintaining healthy relationships. Spending time with our loved ones, sharing experiences, and creating memories together can enrich our lives in profound ways.

The environment we live in also impacts our well-being. A clean, organized and pleasant environment can improve our mood and productivity. Spending time outdoors, in contact with nature, can be revitalizing and relaxing. Creating a space in our home that reflects our personality and makes us feel comfortable can significantly contribute to our well-being.

Finally, wellness is also about personal growth and self-acceptance. Setting goals, learning new things, and working on our personal development helps us feel fulfilled and satisfied with our lives. Accepting ourselves as we are, with our strengths and weaknesses, and treating ourselves with kindness and respect is essential to our happiness and well-being.

In short, wellness is a continuous journey of self-care and balance. By focusing on physical, emotional and mental health, we can live a fuller and more satisfying life. This book will guide you through the different aspects of well-being, offering you practical advice and strategies to improve your quality of life. Remember that every small positive change you make can have a big impact on your overall well-being. Let's start this journey towards a life of well-being together!

The Mind and Body in Harmony

The balance between mind and body is essential to achieve a state of comprehensive well-being. When we think about our health, we often focus only on the physical aspect, but mental and emotional health are equally important. The mind and body are interconnected; What affects one inevitably affects the other. To live a full and healthy life, it is crucial to understand this connection and work to keep both aspects in harmony.

Imagine your body as a car and your mind as the driver. For a safe and enjoyable trip, the driver must be alert, calm and in control, and the car must be in good working order. If the driver is stressed or distracted, the trip can become dangerous, even if the car is in perfect condition. Likewise, if the car has mechanical problems, the ride will be difficult, even if the driver is in top shape. The key is to ensure that both the mind and body are aligned and working together efficiently.

Stress is a clear example of how the mind and body can influence each other. When we are under stress, our body responds by releasing hormones such as cortisol and adrenaline. These hormones prepare the body for a "fight or flight" response, which can be helpful in emergency situations, but if stress becomes chronic, it can have negative effects on our health. Physical symptoms of stress can include headaches, digestive problems, muscle tension, and sleep problems. At the same time, stress can affect our mental health, causing anxiety, depression, and difficulty concentrating.

One way to maintain harmony between mind and body is through the regular practice of meditation and mindfulness. These techniques help us be present in the moment, reduce stress and improve our mental health. Meditation can be as simple as sitting in a quiet place and focusing on your breathing. As we breathe in and out slowly, we allow ourselves to let go of worries and focus on the here and now. Mindfulness, for its part, involves being aware of our thoughts, emotions and bodily sensations without judging them. By practicing these techniques, we can reduce our body's reaction to stress and improve our mental health.

Physical exercise also plays a vital role in maintaining balance between mind and body.

Regular physical activity not only strengthens our body, but also releases endorphins, the happiness hormones, which improve our mood and reduce stress. It is not necessary to do intensive training to obtain these benefits. Simple activities like walking, swimming, dancing, or yoga can be very effective. Exercise can also improve sleep quality, which is essential for mental and physical health.

Food is another crucial factor in the mind-body connection. A balanced and nutritious diet provides the necessary nutrients for our body to function properly and our mind to remain alert and positive. Foods rich in omega-3s, such as salmon and walnuts, can improve brain health and reduce symptoms of depression. Fresh fruits and vegetables, packed with vitamins and minerals, can boost our energy levels and improve our mood. Avoiding processed foods and refined sugars can prevent energy spikes and dips that can negatively impact our mental health.

Adequate sleep is essential to maintain harmony between mind and body. During sleep, our body repairs itself and our mind processes the day's experiences. Lack of sleep can lead to physical health problems, such as a weakened immune system, and mental health problems, such as irritability and difficulty concentrating. Establishing a regular sleep routine and creating a relaxing sleeping environment can improve the quality of our sleep and, consequently, our overall well-being.

Personal relationships also play an important role in the mind-body connection. Having positive, supportive relationships can improve our mental and physical health. Sharing our thoughts and feelings with friends and family helps us release stress and feel understood and supported. On the other hand, toxic relationships can increase stress and negatively affect our health. It is important to surround ourselves with people who give us positive energy and help us grow.

Finally, self-care is essential to maintain harmony between mind and body. This includes taking time to relax, do things we enjoy, and take care of our emotional health. Activities such as reading, listening to music, spending time in nature or practicing a hobby can help us recharge our energy and improve our overall well-being.

In conclusion, the connection between mind and body is powerful and fundamental to our well-being. By taking care of both our mental and physical health, we can live a more balanced and satisfying life. This book will provide you with the tools and strategies necessary to maintain this harmony and improve your quality of life. Remember that every small step you take towards mind-body balance will bring you closer to a fuller, healthier life. Let's continue this path together towards a life of well-being!

Healthy Eating for Well-being

Healthy eating is one of the most important pillars to achieve and maintain well-being. What we eat not only affects our physical health, but also our energy, mood and ability to cope with everyday life. A balanced and nutritious diet can be the difference between feeling exhausted and listless or vibrant and full of life. Eating well is one of the best investments we can make in ourselves.

Let's start with the basic principles of a balanced diet. A healthy diet includes a variety of foods from all the major groups: fruits, vegetables, proteins, whole grains, and dairy or their alternatives. Each food group provides different essential nutrients that our body needs to function properly. Fruits and vegetables, for example, are rich in vitamins, minerals and fiber, which help keep our digestive system healthy and our immune system strong.

Proteins are essential for the repair and construction of tissues in our body. Healthy protein sources include lean meats, fish, eggs, legumes and nuts. Whole grains, such as brown rice, quinoa, and oats, provide sustained energy thanks to their fiber and nutrient content. Dairy and its alternatives, such as milk, yogurt and plant milks, are important for bone health due to their calcium and vitamin D content.

A crucial part of healthy eating is moderation. It's not about eliminating all the foods we enjoy, but rather finding a balance. We can enjoy pizza or ice cream from time to time, as long as they do not become the basis of our diet. The key is to eat a variety of foods and not overdo any one in particular. Eating in appropriate portions and paying attention to our body's hunger and satiety signals can help us maintain that balance.

Meal planning can be a very useful tool for maintaining a balanced diet. Taking the time to plan our meals and snacks can help us make sure we are getting all the nutrients we need. We can start by making a shopping list that includes a variety of fruits, vegetables, proteins and whole grains. Preparing homemade meals instead of relying on processed foods or fast food allows us to control ingredients and make healthier choices.

Hydration is also a fundamental part of healthy eating. Our body is largely made up of water, and we need to stay well hydrated for it to function properly. Water helps transport nutrients throughout the body, eliminates waste, and keeps our cells hydrated. Drinking enough water throughout the day is crucial for our energy and overall well-being. In addition to water, we can hydrate ourselves with herbal infusions, water with lemon and other sugar-free drinks.

It is also important to be aware of the foods that we should limit. Foods high in refined sugars, saturated fats and sodium can have negative effects on our health if consumed in excess. Refined sugars, present in many sweets, soft drinks, and processed foods, can cause energy spikes and dips that affect our mood and concentration. Saturated and trans fats, found in fried foods and some baked goods, can increase the risk of heart disease. Excess sodium, common in processed foods and fast food, can contribute to hypertension.

Another way to promote healthy eating is to listen to our body and be aware of our needs and desires. Sometimes we eat for emotional reasons, such as stress or boredom, rather than hunger. Practicing mindfulness when eating can help us recognize when we are truly hungry and when we are eating for other reasons. This means paying attention to our food, savoring each bite, and being present at the time of eating.

Healthy eating can also be fun and creative. Experimenting with new recipes, trying different foods, and enjoying meal preparation can make eating well an enjoyable experience. Cooking at home allows us to be creative and adapt meals to our tastes and needs. Additionally, involving the family in meal preparation can be a great way to spend time together and teach children about the importance of a balanced diet.

We must not forget that food is only one part of well-being. Combining a healthy diet with regular exercise, good sleep and stress management can further enhance our efforts to live a balanced and healthy life. Everything is interconnected; Taking care of our diet can have a positive effect on other aspects of our lives.

In conclusion, a healthy diet is essential for our general well-being. By choosing a variety of nutritious foods, staying hydrated, limiting processed foods, and being mindful of our needs and wants, we can improve our physical and mental health. This chapter has given you an overview of how a balanced diet can transform your life. In the following chapters, we will explore more strategies and tips to maintain and improve your well-being. Enjoy a life with well-being and good nutrition!

The importance of Hydration

Staying well hydrated is essential for our overall well-being. Water is essential for almost all of our body's functions. From regulating body temperature to eliminating toxins, facilitating digestion and keeping skin healthy, water is vital. However, we often underestimate its importance and do not drink enough water throughout the day.

Our body is largely made up of water, around 60%. This shows us how crucial water is to our functioning. Every cell, tissue and organ depends on water to work properly. For example, water helps transport nutrients and oxygen to cells, enables food digestion, lubricates joints, and protects sensitive organs and tissues. Without adequate hydration, all of these processes can be affected.

One of the main benefits of staying hydrated is regulating body temperature. When we exercise, are exposed to heat, or are simply moving, our body sweats to cool itself. This transpiration is essential, but it also means that we are losing water. If we do not replace that water loss, we can become dehydrated. Dehydration can cause fatigue, dizziness, and other health problems.

Drinking enough water helps maintain a stable body temperature and allows us to feel more comfortable and energetic.

Water also plays a crucial role in digestion. It helps break down food, allowing our body to absorb nutrients more efficiently. Additionally, water is essential for preventing constipation as it keeps the intestines functioning properly. Drinking enough water makes it easier for food to pass through the digestive tract and helps waste to be eliminated effectively. If we are not well hydrated, we can experience digestive problems and discomfort.

Proper hydration is also key to maintaining healthy skin. Our skin is the largest organ in the body and needs water to stay elastic and soft. When we are dehydrated, our skin can become dry and prone to wrinkles. Drinking enough water can improve the appearance of our skin, making it look fresher and more radiant. Additionally, well-hydrated skin is more resistant to injury and heals more quickly.

The brain also benefits greatly from hydration. About 75% of our brain is water, and staying hydrated is essential for optimal cognitive function. Dehydration can negatively affect our concentration, memory and mood. Studies have shown that even mild dehydration can decrease cognitive performance. Drinking water regularly helps us stay focused, alert and in a better mood.

For many people, the question is how much water they should drink. The amount of water we need can vary depending on age, gender, physical activity level, and climate. A common recommendation is to drink at least eight glasses of water a day, which is equivalent to about two liters. However, some people may need more, especially if they are very active or live in hot climates. A good way to ensure that we are well hydrated is to pay attention to our body. Thirst is a clear sign that we need water, but we can also look at the color of our urine: if it is clear or pale yellow, we are generally well hydrated.

Not only water counts for our daily fluid intake. We can also hydrate ourselves through other liquids and foods. Fruits and vegetables, such as watermelon, cucumber and oranges, have a high water content and can contribute to our hydration. Herbal infusions, teas, and soups are also good options. However, it is important to limit drinks that can dehydrate us, such as those containing caffeine and alcohol. Although they may seem refreshing, they can have a diuretic effect and increase fluid loss.

Another important aspect of hydration is maintaining a regular routine. Drinking large amounts of water at once is not as effective as drinking small amounts throughout the day. Keeping a water bottle on hand and drinking from it frequently can help us make sure we are getting enough water. It's also helpful to set reminders to drink water, especially if we're busy and it's easy to forget.

Proper hydration is especially important during exercise. When we exercise, we lose water through sweat and we need to replace those fluids to maintain our performance and avoid dehydration. Drinking water before, during and after exercise can help us stay hydrated and recover faster. It's also important to pay attention to electrolytes, which are essential minerals that we lose through sweat. In intense or long-duration physical activities, a sports drink can help replenish both water and electrolytes.

In conclusion, hydration is essential for our general well-being. Drinking enough water and staying hydrated helps us regulate body temperature, improve digestion, keep skin healthy, and support brain function. By paying attention to our fluid intake and making hydration a daily priority, we can significantly improve our health and well-being. This chapter has explored the importance of hydration and how to stay well hydrated. In the following chapters, we will continue to explore more essential aspects of living a life of well-being. Let's continue hydrating and enjoying a full and healthy life!

Physical Exercise and Wellness

Physical exercise is essential for our general well-being. It not only improves our physical health, but also has a positive impact on our mental and emotional health. Exercising regularly can help us feel more energetic, improve our mood, and increase our quality of life. Plus, it's not just about spending hours in the gym; Any type of physical activity can have great benefits.

Let's start by understanding how exercise affects our body. When we move, our heart pumps more blood, which improves circulation and helps oxygenate our muscles and organs. This strengthens the heart and lungs, and improves our resistance. Additionally, regular exercise can help control weight, reduce the risk of chronic diseases such as diabetes and heart disease, and improve our bone and muscle health.

Exercise also plays a crucial role in mental health. When we exercise, our body releases endorphins, known as the happy hormones. These endorphins act as natural pain relievers and mood elevators, making us feel happier and more relaxed. Additionally, exercise can reduce levels of the stress hormone cortisol, helping us better manage stress and anxiety. This means that exercising regularly can be a powerful tool in improving our emotional well-being.

One of the best things about exercise is that there are many ways to do it, and we can find something we really enjoy. It is not necessary to join a gym if we do not like that. Walking, running, swimming, biking, dancing, practicing yoga, or even playing with the kids in the park are great ways to stay active. The key is to find an activity that we like and that we can do consistently. When we enjoy what we do, we are more likely to stick with it for the long term.

Exercise not only benefits the body and mind, but it can also be a great way to socialize and connect with others. Participating in team sports, group fitness classes, or simply going for a walk with a friend can make exercise more fun and allow us to build social relationships. These connections can provide emotional support and motivation, which is essential to our overall well-being.

Establishing an exercise routine may seem challenging at first, especially if we are not used to being active. However, it is important to start small and gradually increase the amount of activity. Even small amounts of exercise can make a big difference. For example, start with a 10-minute walk a day and increase the time and intensity over time. Consistency is key, and every little step counts.

It is also important to listen to our body and not overdo it. Exercise should be challenging, but should not cause pain or injury. If we experience pain, dizziness or difficulty breathing, it is important to stop and seek medical advice if necessary. Additionally, incorporating warm-up and cool-down exercises into our routine can help prevent injuries and improve flexibility.

Exercise not only helps us stay fit, but it can also improve our quality of sleep. Regular physical activity can help us fall asleep faster and enjoy deeper, more restful sleep. Good sleep is essential for muscle recovery and mental well-being, creating a positive cycle where exercise and good sleep reinforce each other.

It's also helpful to set realistic and achievable goals when it comes to exercise. These goals can be as simple as walking 30 minutes a day, completing a 5K run, or improving at a specific activity, such as swimming or biking. By achieving these goals, we feel motivated and have a sense of accomplishment that can boost our confidence and overall well-being.

Exercise can also be a great way to connect with nature. Going for a walk or run in a park, hiking in the mountains or swimming in the sea allows us to enjoy fresh air and natural beauty. Nature has a calming effect on our minds and can further enhance the benefits of exercise.

In conclusion, physical exercise is an essential part of well-being. It helps us stay healthy, improves our mood, reduces stress and allows us to enjoy life more. Finding an activity we enjoy and making it part of our daily routine can have a significant impact on our quality of life. No matter what our age or fitness level, we can always find ways to be more active and enjoy the benefits of exercise. This chapter has explored how exercise can improve our well-being, and in the following chapters, we will continue to explore more aspects essential to living a life of well-being. Get moving and enjoy a healthier, happier life!

Restful Sleep

Restful sleep is one of the fundamental pillars for our general well-being. Getting a good night's sleep not only helps us feel rested and energized the next day, but it also has a profound impact on our physical and mental health. Good sleep is essential for the optimal functioning of our body and mind. However, many people underestimate the importance of sleep and, as a result, suffer the consequences of not getting enough sleep or not having good quality sleep.

Let's start by understanding why sleep is so crucial. While we sleep, our body carries out a series of vital processes. For example, tissue repair occurs, the immune system is strengthened, and the memories and learnings of the day are consolidated. Our brain also benefits from sleep, as it eliminates accumulated toxins and prepares for a new day of activity. Without adequate sleep, these processes are disrupted, which can lead to a variety of health problems.

One of the most immediate effects of not sleeping well is the feeling of fatigue and lack of energy. When we don't get enough sleep, it's hard to concentrate, make decisions, and be productive. Lack of sleep can also affect our mood, making us feel irritable, anxious or even depressed. Over time, sleep deprivation can increase your risk of developing chronic diseases such as hypertension, diabetes, and heart disease. Additionally, it can weaken our immune system, making us more susceptible to infections.

To improve the quality of our sleep, it is important to establish a regular sleep routine. This means going to bed and getting up at the same time every day, even on weekends. Our body has an internal clock, known as the circadian rhythm, that regulates our sleep and wake cycles. By maintaining a consistent routine, we can synchronize our internal clock and improve the quality of our sleep. It is also helpful to create a relaxing environment before sleeping. This may include activities such as reading a book, taking a hot bath, or practicing meditation. Avoiding the use of electronic devices at least an hour before bedtime is also crucial, as the blue light they emit can interfere with the production of melatonin, the sleep hormone.

Diet also plays an important role in sleep quality. Eating heavy or spicy foods right before bed can cause discomfort and make it difficult to sleep. Instead, it is better to opt for a light dinner and consume foods that promote sleep, such as bananas, almonds, or a glass of warm milk. These foods contain nutrients that can help you relax and fall asleep more easily. It's also important to limit caffeine and alcohol, as both can interfere with sleep. Caffeine, found in coffee, tea, and many soft drinks, is a stimulant that can keep us awake if consumed late in the day. Alcohol, although it may make us feel sleepy at first, can disrupt sleep during the night and decrease the quality of rest.

The environment we sleep in also has a big impact on our ability to rest well. A dark, cool, and quiet bedroom is ideal for promoting sleep. Using blackout curtains to block light, keeping the room temperature cool, and using earplugs or a white noise machine can help create an environment conducive to sleep. A comfortable mattress and pillow are also essential. If we don't feel comfortable in bed, we are likely to wake up frequently during the night. Investing in a good bed can make a big difference in the quality of our sleep.

Regular exercise can also improve sleep quality. Physical activity helps reduce stress and anxiety, which can make it easier to sleep. However, it is important not to do intense exercise right before bed, as this can have the opposite effect and make it difficult to sleep. Instead, it is best to exercise in the morning or afternoon. Activities such as yoga or a quiet evening walk can be particularly beneficial for relaxing and preparing for sleep.

Stress management is another crucial aspect of achieving restful sleep. Stress and anxiety can keep us awake at night, ruminating over the day's problems and worries. Developing stress management techniques, such as meditation, deep breathing, or journaling, can help us release tension and prepare our minds to rest. Establishing a relaxation routine before bed can be especially helpful. This could include reading a book, listening to soft music, or practicing breathing exercises.

It is also important to know when to seek professional help if we are having trouble sleeping. If we are experiencing chronic insomnia or if lack of sleep is seriously affecting our daily lives, it may be helpful to speak with a doctor or sleep specialist. They can help us identify any underlying problems and offer specific solutions to improve our sleep.

In conclusion, restful sleep is essential for our overall well-being. Sleeping well improves our physical, mental and emotional health. By establishing a regular sleep routine, creating an environment conducive to rest, maintaining a proper diet, exercising regularly and managing stress, we can significantly improve the quality of our sleep. This chapter has explored the importance of sleep and how we can achieve a restful rest. In the following chapters, we will continue to explore more essential aspects of living a life of well-being. Sweet dreams and a healthier, happier life!

Stress Management

Stress management is essential to leading a life of well-being. Stress is a natural response of the body to challenging or threatening situations. Although in small doses it can be beneficial, motivating us to act and confront problems, chronic stress can have negative effects on our physical and mental health. Therefore, learning to manage stress effectively is key to our well-being.

Let's start by understanding what stress is. When we face a stressful situation, our body goes into a "fight or flight" state. This means that hormones such as cortisol and adrenaline are released, which increase our heart rate, make us breathe faster and prepare our muscles for action. This response is useful in situations of immediate danger, but when we are constantly stressed, our body remains in this state of alert, which can be harmful.

Chronic stress can affect our health in many ways. It can cause headaches, digestive problems, insomnia, and fatigue. It can also weaken our immune system, making us more susceptible to illness. On an emotional level, stress can lead to anxiety, depression and irritability. That's why it's important to find ways to reduce stress and manage it effectively.

One of the most effective ways to manage stress is by practicing deep breathing. When we are stressed, we tend to breathe shallowly, which can increase our anxiety. Practicing deep breathing can help calm the nervous system and reduce stress. Try inhaling deeply through your nose, filling your lungs with air, and then exhale slowly through your mouth. Repeat this process several times until you feel more relaxed.

Meditation is another powerful tool for stress management. Meditation involves focusing on the present and letting go of worries about the past and future. There are many forms of meditation, but a simple technique is to sit in a quiet place, close your eyes, and focus on your breathing. If your mind starts to wander, simply return your attention to your breathing. Practicing meditation for a few minutes each day can have a big impact on your stress level.

Physical exercise is also a great way to reduce stress. When we exercise, our body releases endorphins, which are hormones that make us feel good. Regular exercise can improve our mood, increase our energy and help combat stress. It is not necessary to do intense training; Activities such as walking, swimming or practicing yoga can be very beneficial.

In addition to exercise, maintaining an overall healthy lifestyle can help manage stress. This includes eating a balanced diet, getting enough sleep, and avoiding excessive caffeine and alcohol consumption. Good nutrition and adequate sleep can improve our ability to cope with stress and keep us in a positive state of mind.

Leisure time and recreational activities are also important for stress management. Doing things you enjoy, such as reading, listening to music, painting, or spending time with friends and family, can help you relax and disconnect from daily worries. Spending time on your hobbies and recreational activities can give you a break from stress and make you feel more balanced and happy.

Another useful stress management strategy is learning to say "no." Many times we feel stressed because we take on too many responsibilities and commitments. Learning to set limits and not overload ourselves with tasks can help us reduce stress. It is not necessary to say "yes" to everything; It's okay to prioritize our well-being and take time for ourselves.

Organization and time management can also be a great help. Stress often comes from feeling overwhelmed by the amount of things we have to do. Making a to-do list, setting priorities, and breaking down big projects into smaller steps can make our responsibilities more manageable. Plus, taking regular breaks throughout the day can help us stay focused and avoid burnout.

Talking about our worries with someone we trust can be very liberating. Whether it's a friend, family member, or therapist, sharing our feelings and receiving support can help us see things from a different perspective and find solutions to our problems. We don't have to face stress alone; Seeking support is an important part of stress management.

Humor can also be an effective tool to combat stress. Laughing and finding the funny side of situations can help us relax and see things in a more positive way. Watching a funny movie, reading a funny book, or simply spending time with people who make us laugh can lift our spirits and reduce stress.

Finally, it is important to remember that stress management is an ongoing process. There is no one-size-fits-all solution that works for everyone, and what works for one person may not be effective for another. It is important to try different strategies and find the ones that best suit us. It is also important to be patient with ourselves and recognize that it is okay to have difficult days. The important thing is to continue practicing self-care and do the best we can to manage stress.

In conclusion, stress management is essential for our well-being. Through deep breathing, meditation, exercise, a healthy lifestyle, leisure time, organization, social support and humor, we can reduce stress and improve our quality of life. This chapter has explored various strategies for managing stress, and in the following chapters, we will continue to explore more aspects essential to living a life of well-being. Adopt these practices and enjoy a more balanced and happy life!

Mental and Emotional Health

Mental and emotional health is a crucial component of our overall well-being. It is not just about the absence of mental illness, but the presence of positive thoughts, feelings and behaviors that allow us to manage stress, relate well to others and enjoy life. Just as we take care of our body, it is essential to take care of our mind and our emotions.

To begin with, let's understand what mental health is. Mental health includes our emotional, psychological and social well-being. It affects how we think, feel and act. It also determines how we handle stress, relate to others, and make decisions. Good mental health does not mean that we never experience emotional problems. We all face challenges, but a person with good mental health can handle these challenges effectively.

Self-esteem is a fundamental part of mental health. Having good self-esteem means having a positive view of ourselves, valuing ourselves and feeling confident in our abilities. Self-esteem is not something you have or don't have; It can be worked on and improved over time. One way to do this is by practicing self-compassion, treating ourselves with the same kindness and understanding that we would offer a close friend. Instead of being critical of ourselves for our mistakes, we can recognize that no one is perfect and that everyone makes mistakes.

Healthy relationships are also vital for our mental and emotional health. Having strong connections with friends, family, and peers can provide us with emotional support and a sense of belonging. It is important to surround ourselves with people who make us feel good, who support us and who value us. Toxic relationships, on the other hand, can drain our energy and negatively affect our mental health. Sometimes, it is necessary to set limits and distance ourselves from people or situations that hurt us.

Managing emotions is another essential skill for mental health. We all experience a range of emotions, from joy to sadness, anger and fear. It is important to recognize and accept our emotions instead of repressing or ignoring them. We can learn to manage our emotions in a healthy way, expressing them appropriately and looking for constructive ways to deal with them.

For example, talking to someone we trust, writing in a journal, or engaging in creative activities like art or music can help us process our emotions.

Self-care is a key aspect of mental health. Taking time for ourselves, doing things that we enjoy and that relax us, can improve our emotional well-being. Self-care can be as simple as taking a walk outside, reading a good book, taking a relaxing bath, or taking up a hobby. It is also important to take care of our body, since physical and mental health are interconnected. Eating a balanced diet, exercising regularly and getting enough sleep are essential to maintaining good mental health.

Practicing gratitude can have a positive impact on our emotional health. Taking a few minutes each day to reflect on the things we are grateful for can help us focus on the positive and reduce stress and anxiety. Keeping a gratitude journal, in which we write down three things we are grateful for each day, can be a simple but powerful practice for improving our emotional well-being.

The search for purpose and meaning in life is also essential for our mental health. Having goals and objectives that motivate us and give us a sense of direction can provide us with a deep sense of satisfaction and happiness. It doesn't have to be something great; It can be something as simple as learning a new skill, helping others, or following a passion. The important thing is that we feel committed and that our actions have a purpose.

Resilience is the ability to bounce back from adversity and challenges. Developing resilience is crucial to maintaining good mental health. Resilience does not mean that difficulties do not affect us, but that we have the ability to face and overcome them. We can develop resilience by building a support network, maintaining a positive attitude, being flexible and learning from our experiences.

Seeking help when we need it is a fundamental part of taking care of our mental health. There is no shame in asking for help. If we feel overwhelmed, sad or anxious for a long period of time, talking to a mental health professional, such as a psychologist or counselor, can be very beneficial. They can provide us with tools and strategies to manage our emotions and improve our well-being.

Mindfulness, or full attention, is another practice that can improve our mental health. Mindfulness involves being present in the moment, without judging our experiences. Practicing mindfulness can help us reduce stress, improve our concentration, and increase our self-awareness. We can practice mindfulness through meditation, conscious breathing, or simply paying attention to our daily activities with full awareness.

In conclusion, mental and emotional health is essential for our overall well-being. By caring for our self-esteem, maintaining healthy relationships, managing our emotions, practicing self-care, seeking gratitude, finding purpose, developing resilience, and seeking help when we need it, we can significantly improve our mental and emotional health. This chapter has explored various strategies to take care of our mental health, and in the following chapters, we will continue to explore more essential aspects of living a life of well-being. Let's take care of our minds and our emotions to enjoy a happier and fuller life!

Healthy Relationships

Healthy relationships are essential to our well-being. Not only do they provide us with emotional support, but they also contribute to our happiness and sense of belonging. Having positive relationships with friends, family, and colleagues can enrich our lives in many ways. However, building and maintaining healthy relationships requires effort and attention.

To start, it's important to understand what makes a relationship healthy. Healthy relationships are based on mutual respect, trust and open communication. In a healthy relationship, both individuals feel valued and heard. This means that you respect each other's opinions and feelings, even if you don't always agree. Trust is essential because without it, it is difficult to feel safe and comfortable in a relationship. Open communication means that you can both express your thoughts and feelings honestly and without fear of being judged.

Effective communication is the foundation of any healthy relationship. This involves not only speaking, but also active listening. When someone is talking to us, it is important to pay attention, ask questions, and show genuine interest in what they are saying. Active listening helps strengthen the connection and avoid misunderstandings. Additionally, it is crucial to be clear and direct when expressing our own needs and feelings. Avoiding confrontation can lead to built-up resentments, so it's best to address issues head-on, but in a respectful manner.

Empathy also plays a crucial role in healthy relationships. Empathy is the ability to put yourself in someone else's shoes and understand their feelings and perspectives. Practicing empathy helps us be more understanding and build stronger relationships. When we show empathy, we show the other person that we care and that we are willing to support them. This can strengthen the trust and emotional bond between both of you.

Quality time is another important aspect of healthy relationships. Spending time with the people we care about, whether it's spending time together, talking on the phone, or simply sending a message to see how they are doing, can strengthen our relationships. It's not about the amount of time, but the quality of time we spend together. Doing activities that you both enjoy, such as watching a movie, going for a walk, or cooking together, can help create positive memories and strengthen your connection.

Respect for individuality is also crucial in a healthy relationship. Although it is important to spend time together, it is also essential to respect each other's space and independence. Each person needs time for themselves and to follow their own interests and passions. Respecting this and supporting each other in their individual activities can strengthen the relationship and avoid the feeling of being trapped or dependent.

Resolving conflicts constructively is essential to maintaining healthy relationships. In any relationship, it is normal for disagreements and conflicts to arise. The key is how we handle these conflicts. Instead of resorting to personal attacks or evasion of the problem, it is important to approach conflicts with a solution-oriented attitude. Finding common ground, compromising, and finding solutions that are mutually acceptable can help resolve conflicts positively. Remembering that you are on the same team and that the goal is to strengthen the relationship can change the way you deal with disagreements.

Forgiveness is an essential part of healthy relationships. We all make mistakes, and sometimes, we can hurt those we love, even if it is not intentional. Learning to forgive and let go of resentments is crucial to maintaining a healthy relationship. Forgiveness does not mean forgetting what happened or justifying negative behavior, but choosing to move forward without carrying the weight of resentment. Forgiveness can free both parties and allow the relationship to grow and strengthen.

Gratitude can also play an important role in healthy relationships. Expressing gratitude and appreciation for the small and big things the other person does can strengthen the bond and increase happiness in the relationship. Taking the time to thank and recognize each other's efforts can make them feel valued and motivated to continue contributing positively to the relationship.

It is also important to know how to recognize the signs of an unhealthy relationship. Toxic relationships can negatively affect our emotional and mental well-being. Some signs of a toxic relationship include controlling, manipulation, disrespect, negative communication, and lack of support. If we find ourselves in a toxic relationship, it is crucial to seek help and consider walking away from that relationship to protect our health and well-being.

Mutual support is a key feature of healthy relationships. Being there for each other in times of need, offering a helping hand, or simply being present can strengthen the bond. Support should not only be emotional, but also practical. Helping with everyday tasks, offering advice or simply listening can make a big difference. Knowing that we have someone to trust and who will support us in difficult times is a source of great comfort and security.

Finally, it is important to remember that healthy relationships require continuous effort. They are not something that is achieved once and then put aside. They require regular maintenance and care. This means continuing to work on communication, showing empathy, spending quality time, and resolving conflicts constructively. It also means being willing to adapt and grow together, accepting that people change over time and that relationships evolve.

In conclusion, healthy relationships are essential to our overall well-being. By building on mutual respect, trust and open communication, and by practicing empathy, spending quality time, respecting individuality, resolving conflict constructively, practicing forgiveness, expressing gratitude, recognizing the signs of a toxic relationship, By providing mutual support and maintaining continuous effort, we can build and maintain relationships that enrich us and make us feel happy and supported. This chapter has explored the key elements of healthy relationships, and in the following chapters, we will continue to explore more aspects essential to living a life of well-being. Let's cultivate positive relationships and enjoy a fuller and happier life!

Food and Moods

What we eat has a significant impact on how we feel. Our diet not only affects our physical health, but also our mood and emotional well-being. The foods we consume can influence our energy levels, our concentration and, above all, our emotions. Understanding the connection between food and mood is crucial to leading a life of well-being.

To start, it is important to understand that our brain needs certain nutrients to function properly. These nutrients come from the foods we eat. For example, carbohydrates, proteins, and healthy fats are essential for optimal brain function. Carbohydrates provide glucose, which is the main source of energy for the brain. Proteins contain amino acids, which are essential for the production of neurotransmitters, the chemicals that transmit signals in the brain. Healthy fats, such as omega-3 fatty acids, are vital for brain structure and function.

Carbohydrates have a direct relationship with our mood. Complex carbohydrates, such as those found in whole grains, fruits and vegetables, release glucose slowly and steadily, providing sustained energy. This helps maintain stable blood sugar levels, which is crucial to avoid sudden mood swings. On the other hand, simple carbohydrates, such as refined sugars and processed foods, can cause rapid spikes and drops in blood sugar levels, which can lead to feeling irritable, tired, and having mood swings.

Proteins also play an important role in regulating mood. Amino acids found in proteins are necessary for the production of neurotransmitters such as serotonin, dopamine, and norepinephrine. Serotonin, often known as the "happy hormone," is essential for regulating mood, sleep, and appetite. Foods rich in tryptophan, an essential amino acid found in turkey, chicken, eggs and dairy products, can help increase serotonin levels in the brain, promoting a feeling of well-being.

Healthy fats are essential for emotional well-being. Omega-3 fatty acids, found in fatty fish such as salmon, walnuts, and chia seeds, are especially important for brain health. Omega-3s help reduce inflammation in the brain and may improve symptoms of depression and anxiety. Incorporating these healthy fats into our diet can contribute to better mental health and a more balanced mood.

Vitamins and minerals also play a crucial role in regulating mood. B complex vitamins, such as B6, B12, and folic acid, are important for neurotransmitter production and brain function. Deficiency of these vitamins can lead to memory problems, fatigue and depression. Foods rich in B vitamins include lean meats, eggs, legumes, and leafy green vegetables. Additionally, minerals such as magnesium, zinc, and iron are essential for brain function. Magnesium, found in nuts, seeds, and leafy green vegetables, can help reduce stress and anxiety. Zinc and iron, found in lean meats, seafood and legumes, are necessary for neurotransmitter production and cognitive function.

Proper hydration is another key to maintaining a good mood. Dehydration can negatively affect our ability to concentrate, increase fatigue and cause irritability. Drinking enough water throughout the day is essential to maintain fluid balance in the body and support optimal brain function. Making sure we drink at least eight glasses of water a day can make a big difference in how we feel.

In addition to specific nutrients, the overall quality of our diet also influences our mood. A balanced diet, rich in fruits, vegetables, whole grains, lean proteins and healthy fats, provides the nutrients necessary for optimal brain and body function. Avoiding processed and sugary foods, which often lack nutrients and can contribute to mood swings and feelings of fatigue, is essential for maintaining good mental and emotional health.

It is important to keep in mind that the relationship between food and mood is not unidirectional. Just as our diet can affect how we feel, our moods can also influence our food choices. For example, when we are stressed or sad, we may be tempted to reach for comfort foods, which are often high in sugar and unhealthy fats. These foods may provide temporary relief, but in the long term they can contribute to feelings of discomfort and health problems.

To improve our relationship with food and our mood, it is useful to adopt conscious eating. This means paying attention to what we eat, how we eat, and why we eat. Mindful eating involves eating slowly, enjoying each bite, and listening to our body's hunger and satiety signals. It also means being aware of how we feel before, during and after eating, and choosing foods that nourish us and make us feel good.

Finally, it is important to remember that each person is unique and what works for one person may not work for another. We may need to experiment with different foods and eating patterns to find what best suits our needs and preferences. Consulting with a nutritionist or health professional can be helpful to receive personalized guidance and ensure we are meeting our nutritional needs.

In conclusion, food plays a crucial role in our moods and emotional well-being. By consuming a balanced diet, rich in essential nutrients such as complex carbohydrates, proteins, healthy fats, vitamins and minerals, and staying well hydrated, we can support our mental and emotional well-being. Adopting mindful eating and paying attention to how food affects us can help us feel better and lead a more balanced and happy life. This chapter has explored the connection between food and mood, and in the following chapters, we will continue to explore more aspects essential to living a life of well-being. Let's eat well to feel good and enjoy a full and healthy life!

The Importance of Free Time

Free time is essential for our well-being and happiness. In a society that values productivity and constant work, we often underestimate the importance of taking a break and spending time on activities we enjoy. However, free time is not only a luxury; It is a vital necessity for our emotional, mental and physical balance.

Free time provides us with an opportunity to disconnect from stress and daily demands. Chronic stress can have negative effects on our health, including sleep problems, anxiety, depression and physical illness. Spending time relaxing and doing activities that we like helps us reduce stress and recharge our energy. When we allow ourselves to rest, our body and mind have the opportunity to recover and renew, making us more resilient and better prepared to face life's challenges.

Furthermore, free time is crucial for our creativity and personal development. When we take a break from work and responsibilities, our minds are free to wander and explore new ideas. Many people find that their best ideas and creative solutions come when they are relaxed and not focused on solving specific problems. Engaging in hobbies and creative activities, such as painting, writing, playing an instrument, or cooking, can stimulate our imagination and give us a sense of accomplishment and satisfaction.

Leisure activities also play an important role in our physical health. Physical exercise, for example, is a great way to spend your free time and has numerous health benefits. Activities such as walking, swimming, cycling or playing sports not only improve our physical condition, but also release endorphins, the hormones of happiness, which improve our mood. Additionally, regular exercise can reduce the risk of chronic diseases, improve sleep quality, and increase our energy.

Free time is also essential to strengthen our social relationships. Spending time with friends and family, without the distractions of work and other responsibilities, allows us to connect in deeper and more meaningful ways. Shared activities, such as playing games, going on hikes, or just talking, can strengthen bonds and create happy memories. Healthy social relationships are essential to our emotional well-being and provide us with a support system in times of need.

The importance of free time also extends to the opportunity to learn and grow. Using free time to explore new interests and learn new skills can enrich our lives and give us a sense of purpose. Learning a new language, taking dance classes, reading books on topics that interest us or traveling to new places are ways to expand our horizons and develop our capabilities. This personal growth contributes to our self-esteem and helps us feel more fulfilled and happy.

It is important to mention that free time should not be seen as a waste of time. On the contrary, it is an investment in our long-term well-being and productivity. When we take time to rest and enjoy, we return to our daily tasks with a clearer and refreshed mind, allowing us to be more efficient and effective in our work and responsibilities.

To make the most of our free time, it is useful to plan and prioritize it. In our busy schedules, it's easy to put free time on the back burner. However, it is essential to reserve specific times for leisure and relaxation activities. This may involve setting clear boundaries between work and personal time, and ensuring that we are not constantly available for work tasks outside of our working hours. Creating a balance between responsibilities and free time is key to maintaining a healthy and balanced life.

It is also important to listen to our body and mind and recognize when we need a break. Ignoring signs of burnout can lead to emotional and physical exhaustion. Taking regular breaks, even if they are brief, during the day can help maintain our energy levels and prevent accumulated stress. Even a few minutes of meditation, deep breathing, or a short walk can make a big difference in how we feel.

Furthermore, it is essential that free time is truly relaxing and enjoyable. It's not just about doing activities that we like, but also about avoiding those that cause us stress or exhaust us. For example, although social media can be a form of entertainment, it can also be a source of stress and negative comparison. It is important to be aware of how we use our free time and choose activities that really make us feel good and relax us.

Finally, it is essential to remember that free time is personal and varies from one person to another. What is relaxing and enjoyable for one person may not be so for another. Some people may find peace in nature, while others may enjoy a social or creative activity more. The important thing is to identify what makes us feel good and make sure to dedicate time to those activities regularly.

In conclusion, free time is an essential part of a well-being life. It allows us to relax, reduce stress, stimulate our creativity, improve our physical health, strengthen our social relationships and grow as individuals. By prioritizing and planning our free time, we can enjoy its many benefits and live a more balanced and happy life. This chapter has explored the importance of free time, and in the following chapters, we will continue to explore more essential aspects of living a life of well-being. Let's take the time to enjoy and take care of ourselves!

Financial Wellbeing

Financial well-being is an essential component of a balanced and happy life. Having our finances in order not only provides us with security and peace of mind, but also allows us to enjoy life without the constant worry about money. However, achieving financial well-being requires planning, discipline, and a clear understanding of our financial goals and priorities.

To start, it's crucial to understand what financial well-being really means. It's not just about earning a lot of money, but about knowing how to manage our income and expenses effectively. This includes having a clear budget, saving for the future, investing wisely, and most importantly, avoiding unnecessary debt. Financial stability gives us the freedom to make decisions without the constant stress of economic insecurity.

The first step towards financial well-being is to create a budget. A budget helps us understand how much money comes in and how much goes out each month. This allows us to see where we are spending too much and where we can cut expenses. To make a budget, write down all your income and then list all your expenses, from the biggest ones like rent or mortgage, to the smallest ones like your daily coffee. By having a clear view of your finances, you can make informed decisions and avoid unnecessary expenses.

Once you have a budget, the next step is to save. Saving money regularly is essential to achieving financial well-being. It's not just about having an emergency fund, although this is very important, but also about saving for long-term goals such as retirement, children's education, or buying a home. A good goal is to save at least 20% of your monthly income. To make it easier, you can automate your savings by automatically transferring a portion of your salary to a savings account each month.

Smart investments are also key to financial well-being. Investing your money allows you to grow it over time. There are many forms of investing, from stocks and bonds to real estate and mutual funds. The key is to diversify your investments to reduce risk and increase the chances of good returns. If you're not sure where to start, consider consulting a financial advisor who can help you create an investment strategy tailored to your goals and risk tolerance.

Another important aspect of financial well-being is avoiding unnecessary debt. Not all debts are bad; Some, like a mortgage to buy a home, can be valuable investments. However, high-interest debt, such as credit card debt, can quickly become a financial burden. It is important to use credit responsibly and pay debts on time to avoid additional interest and fees. If you already have debts, create a plan to pay them off as quickly as possible, starting with those with the highest interest.

Financial education also plays a crucial role in financial well-being. The more you know about how to manage your money, the easier it will be to make wise financial decisions. This may include reading books on personal finance, taking online courses, attending financial workshops, or simply talking to experts in the field. Financial education empowers you to take control of your finances and avoid common mistakes that can cost you dearly in the long term.

Planning for the future is another fundamental piece of financial well-being. This includes not only saving for retirement, but also planning for other important life events, such as children's education, travel, and other personal goals. Use tools like retirement accounts and education savings plans to make sure you're prepared for the future. Additionally, having adequate insurance, such as health insurance, life insurance, and property insurance, can protect you from unexpected expenses and provide peace of mind.

It is also important to consider the importance of living within our means. In an era of consumerism, it is easy to fall into the trap of spending more than we earn. However, this only leads to debt and financial stress. Living within our means means being aware of our spending habits and prioritizing needs over wants. This does not mean that we cannot treat ourselves from time to time, but that we must do it in a planned manner and without compromising our financial stability.

Another aspect of financial well-being is the importance of having an emergency fund. Life is full of unexpected events, and having an emergency fund can be a lifesaver in difficult situations, such as job loss, an unexpected illness, or urgent home repairs. An emergency fund should ideally cover three to six months of living expenses. Having this financial cushion gives us peace of mind and allows us to face unforeseen events without resorting to debt.

Financial well-being also involves having a positive mindset towards money. Often, our emotions and beliefs about money can influence our financial decisions. It is important to develop a healthy relationship with money, seeing saving and investing as opportunities to grow and secure our future, rather than as sacrifices. A positive mindset helps us stay motivated and committed to our financial goals.

Finally, it is important to remember that financial well-being is an ongoing process. It is not about achieving a goal and then forgetting it, but about continuing to manage our finances responsibly throughout our lives. Regularly reviewing our budget, adjusting our goals, and adapting to changes in our circumstances is crucial to maintaining good long-term financial health.

In conclusion, financial well-being is an essential part of a well-being life. By creating a budget, saving regularly, investing wisely, avoiding unnecessary debt, educating ourselves about finances, planning for the future, living within our means, having an emergency fund, and maintaining a positive mindset toward money, we can achieve stability. and financial security. This chapter has explored the key elements of financial well-being, and in the following chapters, we will continue to explore more aspects essential to living a life of well-being. Let's take control of our finances and enjoy a safer and happier life!

Spirituality and Wellbeing

Spirituality is an essential component of well-being that is often overlooked. It's not just about following a specific religion or beliefs, but about finding a sense of purpose and connection in life. Spirituality can take many different forms and mean different things to different people, but at its core, it helps us feel more whole, at peace, and in harmony with ourselves and the world around us.

For many people, spirituality is a source of strength and comfort in difficult times. It gives us a sense of belonging and connection to something larger than ourselves, whether it be a deity, nature, the universe, or a community of people with similar beliefs. This connection helps us face life's challenges with more serenity and confidence, knowing that we are not alone and that there is a deeper purpose to our experiences.

Spirituality also offers us a way to explore and understand our deepest emotions and thoughts. Through spiritual practices such as meditation, prayer, reflection, and time in nature, we can find moments of calm and clarity in the midst of daily chaos. These practices allow us to disconnect from worldly concerns and focus on ourselves, helping us find peace and balance.

One of the most important benefits of spirituality is its ability to reduce stress and anxiety. In a fast-paced and pressure-filled world, finding time to connect with our spiritual side can be a refuge. Meditation, for example, has been scientifically proven to reduce stress levels, improve concentration, and promote a state of general well-being. Prayer and other forms of devotion can also have similar effects, providing a space for gratitude, hope, and inner peace.

Furthermore, spirituality encourages us to live in accordance with our values and principles. By reflecting on what is truly important to us, we can make decisions that are more aligned with our ideals and life purpose. This helps us live in a more authentic and meaningful way, which is essential for our emotional and mental well-being. Living in harmony with our values gives us a sense of satisfaction and helps us avoid the stress and anxiety that can arise from incongruence between our actions and our beliefs.

Spirituality also encourages compassion and love for others. By feeling connected to something bigger than ourselves, we are more likely to treat others with kindness and respect. This not only improves our personal relationships, but also contributes to a sense of community and mutual support. Healthy, meaningful relationships are critical to our well-being, and spirituality helps us cultivate these connections in deeper and more genuine ways.

Exploring spirituality also invites us to be more aware of the present. Many spiritual practices, such as meditation and mindfulness, focus on being present in the moment and appreciating the beauty and simplicity of everyday life. This awareness of the present helps us enjoy life more, reduce stress about future worries, and feel more grateful for what we have. Gratitude, in particular, is a powerful spiritual practice that can transform our perspective and increase our happiness.

It is important to note that spirituality is a deeply personal and unique experience for each individual. There is no right or wrong way to be spiritual. Some people find spirituality in organized religion, while others find it in nature, in artistic practice, in music, in service to others, or in the pursuit of knowledge. The crucial thing is to find what resonates with us and helps us feel more connected and at peace.

For those who do not have an established spiritual practice, it can be helpful to explore different paths and see what speaks to you most. This could include reading books on spirituality, attending religious services, practicing yoga or tai chi, spending time in nature, or simply setting aside a few minutes a day for meditation or reflection. Spiritual exploration is an ongoing and personal journey, and it is important to be patient and open to new experiences.

In short, spirituality is a vital component of well-being that helps us find a sense of purpose, peace, and connection in life. Through spiritual practices, we can reduce stress, live according to our values, cultivate compassion and love for others, and be more aware of the present. Spirituality offers us a way to explore and understand our deepest emotions and thoughts, and provides us with a source of strength and comfort in difficult times. By integrating spirituality into our lives, we can achieve greater well-being and a fuller, more meaningful life.

This chapter has explored the importance of spirituality for well-being, and in the following chapters, we will continue to explore more aspects essential to living a life of well-being. Find your spiritual path and discover how it can enrich your life and provide you with a deep sense of peace and happiness!

Environment and Wellbeing

The environment in which we live and develop has a significant impact on our well-being. Our environment can influence how we feel, how we think and how we act. From the quality of the air we breathe to the organization of our personal space, every aspect of our environment contributes to our physical, mental and emotional well-being. Creating and maintaining a healthy and positive environment is essential to living a full and balanced life.

One of the most important aspects of the environment is air quality. Breathing clean air is essential for our health. Air pollution can cause a number of health problems, from respiratory diseases to cardiovascular problems. Therefore, it is important to take measures to improve the air quality in our homes and workplaces. This may include using air purifiers, keeping windows open to allow ventilation, and avoiding the use of toxic chemicals that can release contaminants into the air. In addition, planting trees and maintaining plants at home can help purify the air and improve the quality of the environment.

The organization and cleanliness of our personal space also plays a crucial role in our well-being.

A messy and dirty space can cause stress, anxiety and difficulty concentrating. Maintaining an orderly and clean environment helps us feel calmer and in control. This doesn't mean everything has to be spotless all the time, but regularly taking time to organize and clean our space can make a big difference in how we feel. Plus, getting rid of things we no longer need or use can create a more spacious and stress-free environment.

Natural light is another important environmental factor that affects our well-being. Exposure to natural light not only improves our mood, it also regulates our circadian rhythm, helping us sleep better and feel more alert and energetic during the day. Trying to spend time outdoors, opening curtains and blinds during the day and, if necessary, using lamps that imitate natural light, can have a positive impact on our well-being.

The colors around us can also influence our mood and well-being. Colors have the power to affect our emotions in different ways. For example, soft, neutral colors like blue and green can have a calming effect, while bright colors like red and yellow can energize us and improve our mood. Choosing colors that make us feel good and that adapt to the different functions of the spaces in our home can contribute to a more harmonious and pleasant environment.

Sound is another aspect of the environment that can affect our well-being. Constant, loud noises can cause stress and affect our ability to concentrate and relax. On the other hand, soft, pleasant sounds, such as calm music, birdsong, or the sound of water, can have a calming and rejuvenating effect. Creating a sound environment that promotes relaxation and concentration can significantly improve our quality of life.

The presence of nature in our environment is also essential for our well-being. Numerous studies have shown that spending time in nature can reduce stress, improve mood, and increase overall feelings of well-being. If we live in an urban area, we can try to incorporate elements of nature into our environment, such as houseplants, container gardens, or aquariums. It is also beneficial to regularly take time to visit parks, gardens and other green spaces where we can connect with nature and enjoy its beauty and serenity.

The temperature and ventilation of our environment are also crucial for our well-being. An environment that is too hot or cold can cause discomfort and affect our health. Maintaining a pleasant and constant temperature, as well as ensuring good ventilation, helps us feel more comfortable and prevent health problems related to extreme temperatures. Using fans, heaters or air conditioning systems properly can help maintain a healthy and comfortable environment.

The furniture and layout of our space can also influence our well-being. A well-designed and comfortable environment can improve our productivity, creativity and overall well-being. Choosing ergonomic furniture that supports good posture, arranging the space in a way that facilitates movement and interaction, and creating areas dedicated to different activities, such as working, relaxing and socializing, can make our environment more functional and pleasant.

Technology also plays an important role in our environment. Although technology can be a valuable tool, its excessive or inappropriate use can negatively affect our well-being. Spending too much time in front of screens can cause eye strain, sleep problems, and increased stress. It's important to set boundaries and take regular breaks from technology to maintain a healthy balance. Creating technology-free spaces, such as rest areas or bedrooms, can help us disconnect and relax.

Finally, the emotional environment of our environment is also crucial for our well-being. A positive and supportive environment helps us feel safe, valued and motivated. This includes surrounding ourselves with people who support us and make us feel good, as well as creating an environment that reflects our values and aspirations. Open and respectful communication, recognition and gratitude, and creating an inclusive and welcoming environment are essential for a healthy emotional environment.

In conclusion, the environment in which we live and develop has a significant impact on our well-being. From air quality to the organization of our space, every aspect of our environment contributes to our physical, mental and emotional well-being. Creating and maintaining a healthy and positive environment is essential to living a full and balanced life. By taking steps to improve our environment, we can enjoy greater peace of mind, happiness and satisfaction in our daily lives. This chapter has explored the importance of the environment for well-being, and in the following chapters, we will continue to explore more aspects essential to living a life of well-being. Create an environment that makes you feel good and enjoy a more harmonious and balanced life!

Nutrition and Detoxification

Nutrition and detoxification are two fundamental aspects to maintain a life of well-being. The way we eat and how we help our body eliminate toxins have a direct impact on our physical, mental and emotional health. In this chapter, we will explore how good nutrition and detoxification practices can help us feel better, have more energy, and live healthier lives.

Let's start with nutrition. Eating healthy not only means choosing nutritious foods, but also understanding how these foods affect our body and mind. A balanced diet should include a variety of essential nutrients, such as proteins, carbohydrates, healthy fats, vitamins and minerals. Each of these nutrients plays a crucial role in maintaining our bodily functions, from building and repairing tissues to providing energy and supporting the immune system.

Proteins are the building blocks of our body. They are present in foods such as lean meats, fish, eggs, legumes and nuts. Eating enough protein is vital for maintaining and repairing muscle tissues, producing enzymes and hormones, and maintaining a healthy immune system.

Additionally, protein helps us feel fuller for longer, which can be useful for weight control.

Carbohydrates are our body's main source of energy. They are found in foods such as fruits, vegetables, whole grains and legumes. It's important to choose complex carbohydrates, which are digested more slowly and provide sustained energy, rather than simple carbohydrates, which can cause rapid blood sugar spikes followed by crashes. Complex carbohydrates also contain fiber, which is essential for healthy digestion.

Healthy fats are equally important for good nutrition. They are found in foods such as avocados, nuts, seeds, olive oil, and fatty fish. These fats are essential for the absorption of fat-soluble vitamins (A, D, E and K), the production of hormones and the protection of our organs. Healthy fats can also help reduce the risk of heart disease and improve brain health.

Vitamins and minerals are micronutrients that our body needs in small quantities but are essential for numerous bodily functions. Fruits and vegetables are excellent sources of these nutrients. Eating a wide variety of colors in our fruits and vegetables ensures that we are getting a full range of vitamins and minerals necessary for our well-being. For example, oranges and other citrus fruits are rich in vitamin C, which strengthens the immune system, while spinach and other leafy greens contain iron, necessary for the production of red blood cells.

In addition to a balanced diet, detoxification is an important process to keep our body clean and functioning optimally. Our body has its own detoxification systems, mainly the liver, kidneys, lungs and skin. However, in the modern world, we are exposed to a large number of toxins through the air we breathe, the food we eat, and the products we use. Helping our body eliminate these toxins can improve our health and well-being.

An effective way to support our body's natural detoxification is to stay well hydrated. Drinking enough water helps the kidneys eliminate toxins through urine. It also keeps the skin hydrated and facilitates digestion. It is recommended to drink at least eight glasses of water a day, although the amount may vary depending on individual needs and activity level.

Eating foods rich in antioxidants is another way to help our body detoxify. Antioxidants are compounds that protect our cells from damage caused by free radicals, which are unstable molecules that can cause chronic diseases. Brightly colored fruits and vegetables, such as berries, grapes, carrots, and peppers, are excellent sources of antioxidants. Incorporating these foods into our daily diet can help our body fight cell damage and stay healthy.

Fibers also play a crucial role in detoxification. Soluble fiber, found in foods such as oats, apples, and legumes, helps lower cholesterol and stabilize blood sugar levels. Insoluble fiber, present in foods such as wheat bran, nuts and green leafy vegetables, facilitates intestinal transit and the elimination of waste from the body. Consuming enough fiber daily is essential to maintaining a healthy and efficient digestive system.

Intermittent fasting is another practice that can support detoxification. This practice involves alternating periods of eating with periods of fasting, allowing the body to rest and focus on cellular repair and the elimination of toxins. Intermittent fasting can have several benefits, such as improving insulin sensitivity, reducing inflammation, and promoting weight loss. However, it is important to do it safely and consult with a health professional before beginning any fasting regimen.

Another way to detoxify is through regular physical exercise. Exercise increases blood circulation and sweating, which helps eliminate toxins through the skin. It also improves digestion and the function of detoxification organs, such as the liver and kidneys. Incorporating physical activity into our daily routine, whether it's walking, running, swimming or practicing yoga, can have a positive impact on our ability to detoxify and our overall health.

Finally, it is important to reduce exposure to toxins as much as possible. This includes choosing organic foods when possible, avoiding cleaning and personal care products with toxic chemicals, and minimizing exposure to environmental contaminants. We can also support detoxification through practices such as deep breathing, which helps eliminate toxins through the lungs, and dry skin brushing, which stimulates circulation and the removal of dead cells.

In short, nutrition and detoxification are essential for our well-being. By eating a balanced diet rich in essential nutrients, staying hydrated, supporting the body's natural detoxification, and reducing exposure to toxins, we can improve our physical, mental, and emotional health. This chapter has explored the importance of nutrition and detoxification for well-being, and in the following chapters, we will continue to explore more essential aspects of living a life of well-being. Let's take care of our body and enjoy a healthier and more balanced life!

Motivation and Personal Growth

Motivation and personal growth are essential components to achieve well-being and a full life. We all have dreams and goals that we want to achieve, but sometimes we encounter obstacles that prevent us from moving forward. Motivation drives us to overcome those obstacles, while personal growth allows us to learn and evolve along the way. In this chapter, we will explore how to stay motivated and committed to our personal growth, in order to achieve our goals and live a more fulfilling life.

Motivation is the force that drives us to act. Without motivation, it is easy to stay stuck and not move forward towards our goals. There are two main types of motivation: intrinsic motivation and extrinsic motivation. Intrinsic motivation comes from within ourselves; It is the desire to do something because we enjoy it or because we believe in its importance. Extrinsic motivation, on the other hand, comes from external factors, such as rewards, recognition, or avoiding negative consequences.

To stay motivated, it is important to identify our sources of intrinsic motivation. What activities are we passionate about? What makes us feel fulfilled and happy? When we align our goals with our passions and values, we are more likely to stay motivated in the long term. For example, if we enjoy helping others, we might pursue goals that involve community service or helping people in need. By doing so, we will find satisfaction in the process, not just the end result.

Setting clear and achievable goals is also crucial to maintaining motivation. Goals give us direction and purpose, and help us measure our progress. It's helpful to break down big goals into smaller, more manageable objectives. This way, we can celebrate our achievements as we go, which reinforces our motivation. For example, if we want to run a marathon, we can start by setting intermediate goals, such as running 5 kilometers, then 10 kilometers, and so on. Every small achievement will bring us closer to our final goal and keep us motivated.

Personal growth is a continuous process of development and improvement. It involves acquiring new knowledge, skills and experiences that help us expand our potential and achieve our goals. Personal growth allows us to adapt to changes, overcome challenges and take advantage of the opportunities presented to us. It is a journey that lasts a lifetime and that leads us to be the best version of ourselves.

One of the keys to personal growth is self-awareness. Knowing ourselves, our strengths and weaknesses, is essential to identify areas in which we need to work and to make the most of our capabilities. Regular reflection, whether through meditation, journaling, or self-assessment, helps us understand our thoughts, emotions, and behaviors. This self-awareness allows us to make more informed and conscious decisions about our growth.

Education and continuous learning are essential components of personal growth. The world is constantly changing, and staying up to date with new knowledge and skills is crucial to adapt and thrive. This doesn't necessarily mean formally going back to school; There are many ways to learn, such as reading books, attending workshops, taking online courses, or simply exploring new interests and hobbies. Learning keeps us curious, open-minded, and prepared to face new challenges.

Resilience is another important quality for personal growth. Life is full of ups and downs, and the ability to bounce back from setbacks is essential to keep moving forward. Resilience allows us to see challenges as opportunities to learn and grow, rather than insurmountable obstacles. We can build resilience by adopting a positive mindset, establishing a strong support network, and practicing self-care.

Self-efficacy, or the belief in our ability to achieve our goals, is essential for motivation and personal growth. Self-efficacy gives us the confidence to face challenges and persevere in the face of difficulties. We can strengthen our self-efficacy by setting and achieving small goals, remembering our past successes, and visualizing our future success. When we believe in ourselves, we are more willing to take risks and strive to achieve our goals.

Social support also plays a crucial role in motivation and personal growth. Surrounding ourselves with people who support and inspire us can make a big difference in our journey to well-being. Friends, family, mentors, and communities can provide motivation, advice, feedback, and encouragement. We should not underestimate the power of social support on our path to personal growth.

Gratitude is another powerful practice that can boost our motivation and personal growth. Taking time to reflect on the things we are grateful for helps us maintain a positive outlook and value our experiences and achievements. Gratitude connects us to the present and allows us to appreciate the progress we have made, which can reinforce our motivation to keep going. Practicing gratitude regularly, whether through a gratitude journal or simply expressing gratitude to others, can have a significant impact on our well-being and growth.

Finally, it is important to remember that personal growth is a unique journey for each individual. There is no single right way to grow and develop. Each of us has our own path and rhythm. It is essential to be patient and compassionate with ourselves, recognize our achievements and learn from our mistakes. Personal growth is not a race, but a continuous journey of self-discovery and improvement.

In summary, motivation and personal growth are essential to achieve well-being and a full life. Motivation drives us to act and overcome obstacles, while personal growth allows us to learn and evolve. By identifying our sources of intrinsic motivation, setting clear goals, developing self-awareness, continually learning, being resilient, strengthening our self-efficacy, seeking social support, and practicing gratitude, we can stay motivated and committed to our personal growth. This chapter has explored the importance of motivation and personal growth for well-being, and in the following chapters, we will continue to explore more aspects essential to living a life of well-being. Stay motivated, continue growing, and enjoy a fuller, more satisfying life!

Technology and Wellbeing

Technology has drastically changed our lives. From smartphones to social media, technology is everywhere and affects almost every aspect of our daily lives. Although technology can offer many advantages and improve our lives in various ways, it can also have negative effects if we do not use it consciously. In this chapter, we will explore how technology can influence our well-being and how we can find a healthy balance in its use.

First, let's look at how technology can improve our well-being. Digital tools offer us access to a large amount of information and resources that can help us live healthier. For example, there are fitness tracking apps that help us stay active, measure our progress, and reach our fitness goals. These apps can remind us when it's time to exercise and offer suggestions to improve our routine. Likewise, there are meditation and relaxation applications that teach us techniques to reduce stress and improve our mental health.

In addition, technology has facilitated access to health and wellness services. Online medical consultations allow people to connect with health professionals without having to travel to a clinic. This is especially useful for those who live in remote areas or have complicated schedules. Online resources also offer us a wide range of information on nutrition, mental health and general well-being, helping us make more informed decisions about our health.

Social media, although often seen as a source of distraction, can also have positive benefits for well-being. They can serve as platforms to connect with friends and family, share experiences, and receive emotional support. Additionally, there are online communities that allow us to find support groups and people with similar interests. These spaces can provide a sense of belonging and support, especially in times of need.

However, excessive use of technology can have negative effects on our well-being. One of the main problems is the dependence on digital devices. Spending too much time in front of a screen can lead to a number of health problems, such as eye strain, headaches, and posture problems. Prolonged exposure to blue light from screens can also affect our sleep, causing insomnia and disturbances in the circadian rhythm. To counteract these effects, it's important to take regular breaks and practice the 20-20-20 rule: every 20 minutes, look at something 20 feet away for at least 20 seconds.

Technology can also affect our mental health. Social media, in particular, can be a source of stress and anxiety. Constant exposure to idealized images and social comparisons can lower our self-esteem and increase feelings of insecurity. Additionally, the pressure to always be connected and available can lead to digital burnout, where we feel overloaded and stressed by the constant communication and demands of technology. Setting limits on social media use and disconnecting from time to time can help mitigate these negative effects.

Another aspect to consider is the impact of technology on our interpersonal relationships. Although technology makes communication easier, it can sometimes make interactions less profound. Face-to-face interaction is essential for developing meaningful connections and maintaining healthy relationships. Spending too much time online can lead to a decrease in the quality of our in-person interactions. It is important to find a balance and make sure to dedicate time to in-person communication and social activities outside of the digital environment.

To achieve balanced and healthy use of technology, it is helpful to set clear boundaries. We can start by creating a schedule for using our devices and ensuring that there are times dedicated to non-technological activities, such as reading a book, playing a sport, or spending time with friends and family. It is also beneficial to designate areas of the house, such as the bedroom, as technology-free zones, to improve sleep quality and reduce the impact of blue light on our rest.

Technology can be a valuable tool for well-being if used in a conscious and balanced way. It is essential to be aware of how the use of technology affects us and make adjustments when necessary to protect our physical, mental and emotional well-being. The key is to find a balance that allows us to enjoy the benefits of technology without sacrificing our health and quality of life.

In conclusion, technology has the potential to improve our well-being by giving us access to useful resources, support and tools. However, it can also have negative effects if not used in a balanced manner. By taking steps to manage our screen time, setting healthy boundaries, and prioritizing in-person interaction, we can enjoy the benefits of technology while maintaining our well-being. This chapter has explored the influence of technology on well-being, and in the following chapters, we will continue to address more aspects essential to living a life of well-being. Use technology consciously and enjoy a balanced and healthy life!